Eggs - Healthy Versatile

A Cookbook to Showcase Them

BY: Ivy Hope

Copyright © 2021 by Ivy Hope

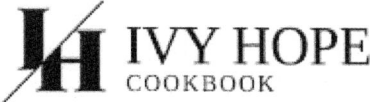

Copyright/License Page

Please don't reproduce this book. It means you are not allowed to make any type of copy (print or electronic), sell, publish, disseminate or distribute. Only people who have written permission from the author are allowed to do so.

This book is written by the author taking all precautions that the content is true and helpful. However, the reader needs to be careful about his/her action. If anything happens due to the reader's actions the author won't be taken as responsible.

Table of Contents

Introduction 5

   Tomatoes, Eggs and Fine Herbs 8

   The Classic and Yummy Egg Salad Sandwich 11

   A Cobb Salad with Chicken 13

   Fun Eggy Dip 15

   Potato Salad with Eggs on top 17

   Multicolored Macaroni Salad with Eggs 19

   Breakfast Idea on Pizza 21

   Deviled Eggs Not So Ordinary 23

   Delicious and Simple Angel Hair Pasta with Eggs and more 25

   Egg Benedict in our Way 27

   Eggs, Cheese and Ham on Sourdough 30

   Weekend Potato and Egg Casserole 32

   Baked Potatoes with Chives, Bacon and Eggs 34

   Crustless Spinach and Cheese Quiche 36

   Omelet Loaded with Meat and Love 39

Eggs in a Creamy Bechamel Sauce 41

Eggs on a Baguette 43

Breakfast or Lunch Egg and Veggie Quesadillas 45

The Egg Drop Soup, just a little Different. 47

Breakfast Burritos Better than at the Restaurant 49

Eggs, Sausage and a whole lot more Casserole 51

Hearty Bacon and Egg Soup 53

Fun Breakfast Idea for Children 55

Chicken Parmesan and Egg Meet 57

Beautiful and Delicious Breakfast Avocados 59

Conclusion 61

About the Author 63

Author's Afterthoughts 64

Introduction

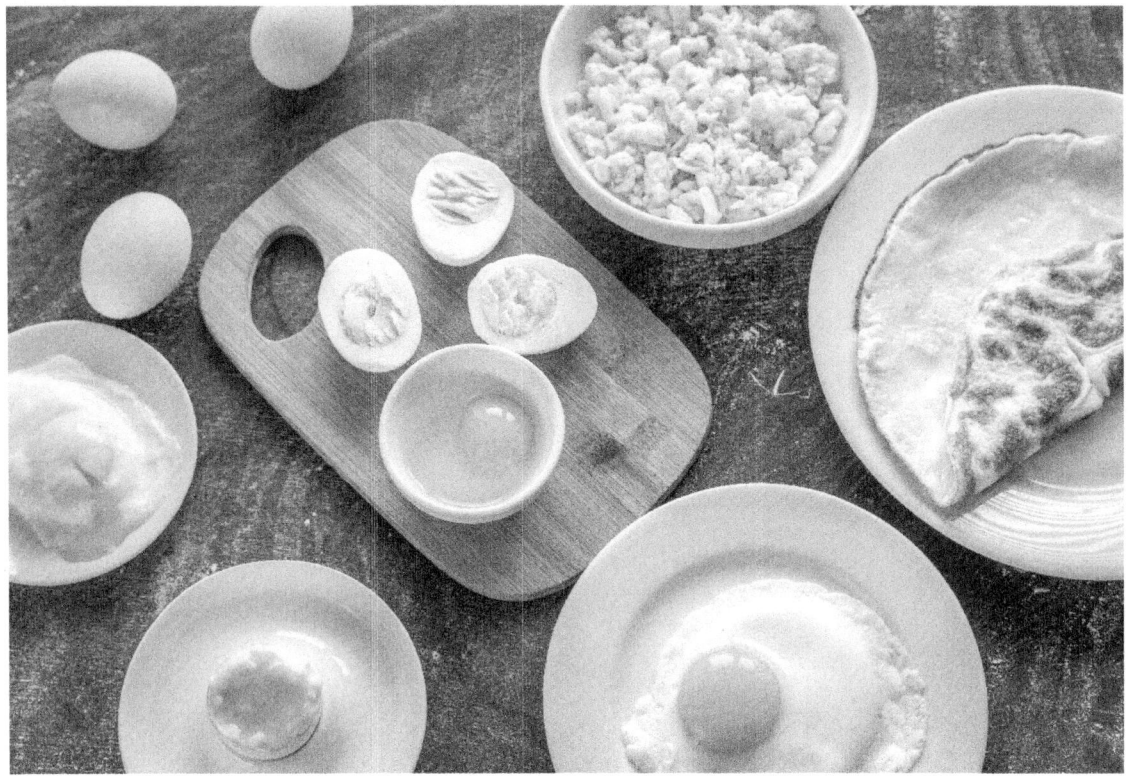

Have you ever heard someone say, I have high cholesterol, or I cannot eat eggs? It is time to clarify the statements. For sure, eggs contain cholesterol, but are they really bad for certain people? We will also inform you of the overall nutritional value and properties that eggs bring to the table.

Nutritional Value

1 egg (medium to large) will provide about 75 calories on average. It will also give you a nice 6 grams of proteins. We will add to this the minerals and vitamins it will offer you: Vitamins A, B12, and Vitamin D.

As far as minerals, you can count magnesium, phosphorus, riboflavin, and zinc, to name just a few.

Here it goes: the yolk of an egg contains 300 mg of cholesterol, which is 2/3 of the recommended intake. Again, there is an ongoing debate on whether it may be too much for certain people, and we will address it below.

Cholesterol debate

Could the cholesterol in egg yolks be more dangerous beneficial for some people? In most cases, moderation is the key once again. Because the yolks contain such a high amount of cholesterol, people who are on a diet to lower their cholesterol level should consume eggs lightly.

There is an important statement you should read. The cholesterol present in eggs is good cholesterol, so it is usually not harmful if you consume only 1 egg a day or less often. Some say that a diet rich in fats can raise your chances for heart diseases much more than eating eggs or add some cholesterol. For any specific medical advice, please consult with your healthcare provider.

However, it is a great idea to eat only egg whites. You can find many different types of egg white beaters or egg white products now in grocery stores. You can even order them at breakfast restaurants now easily instead of the traditional eggs.

Storage and more

If you remember one thing, it is that you should not consume raw eggs. When you add them to baking, you always end up cooking a batter after. Raw eggs can contain salmonella. The dangerous bacteria will, however, be killed when the eggs are cooked. Also, make sure you always store eggs in a cold place as your refrigerator.

Furthermore, refrigerating eggs prevents bacteria and preserves their texture and taste. In the United States, eggs are washed before being sold in stores. It is important to check if your eggs are no cracked before you purchase them.

It is suggested to eat the eggs you purchased within 2 weeks. Not only should you not consume raw eggs but also be careful of cross-contamination. Do not place other ingredients on a surface hosted by raw eggs. Incredibly careful and avoid consuming eggs shells. I know it's typically not used in food, but you could mistakenly leave the shell on your hardboiled eggs or when cracking eggs for preparation. Eggshells can be dirty and unsanitary at times.

Alright, now you know how to safely maneuver eggs and all of the fabulous properties they have. It is time to start using them in your very next recipes.

Tomatoes, Eggs and Fine Herbs

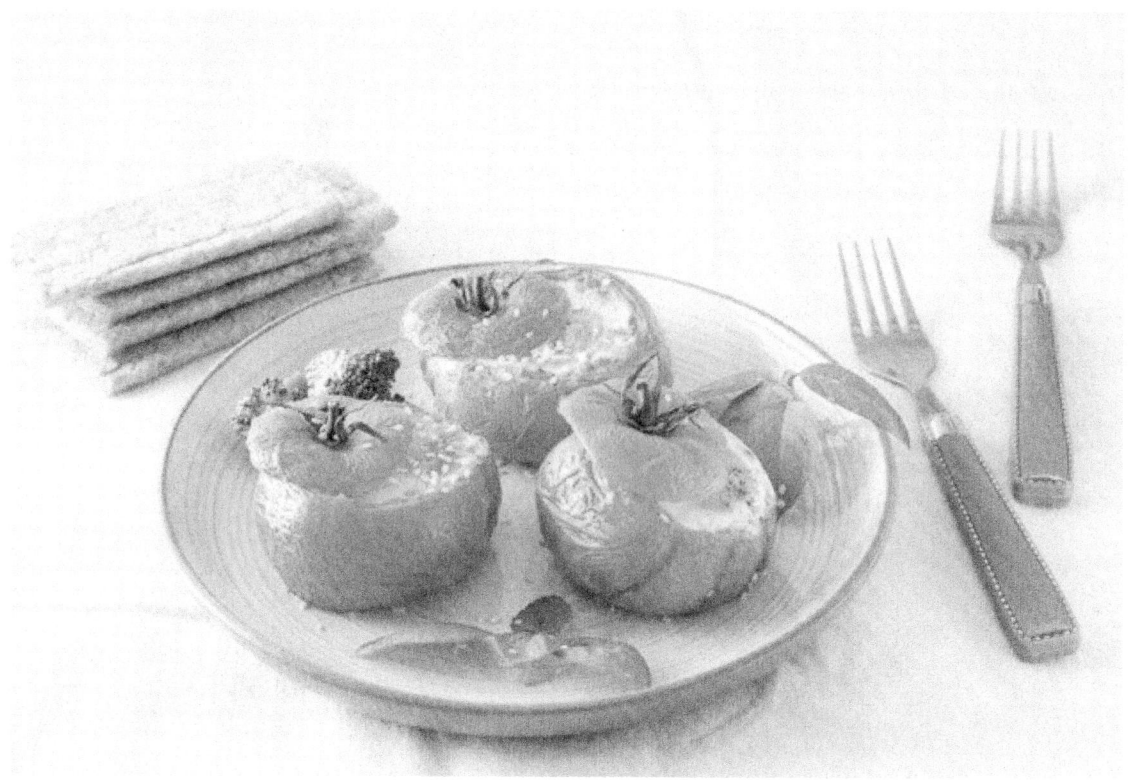

I am a big fan of stuffing vegetables. If you are on a low carbs diet, you must be too. You can stuff avocados, peppers, and why not tomatoes. I think tomatoes, eggs, and cheese go beautifully together. I like to use cream cheese to keep some moisture, as we are going to bake the tomatoes this time.

Serving Size: 4

Cooking Time: 40 Minutes

Ingredients:

- 4 large firm tomatoes
- 1 package cream cheese, room temperature
- 1 tbsp. minced fresh basil
- ¼ diced sweet onion
- ½ tsp. garlic powder
- 8 medium eggs
- Salt, pepper
- Olive oil

Instructions:

1) Preheat the oven to 350 degrees F.

2) Cover a medium sized baking dish with parchment paper. Tomatoes can be messy when cooking, so this will make it much easier to clean up.

3) Next, in a large pan, heat a little oil and cook the basil and onion for 3-4 minutes.

4) After whisking the eggs in a bowl and seasoning with salt and pepper, dump them into the pan.

5) Mix well and cook your scrambled eggs as you love them.

6) Meanwhile, cut your tomatoes in half and scoop some of the flesh out and place in a large mixing bowl.

7) Net, place all tomatoes in the baking dish and brush them with a little olive oil.

8) Place the soft cream cheese in with the tomatoes and once the eggs are cooked, add to the mixture.

9) Then, combine well and stuff each tomato before baking in the oven for 30 minutes or so.

10) Serve with a side salad.

The Classic and Yummy Egg Salad Sandwich

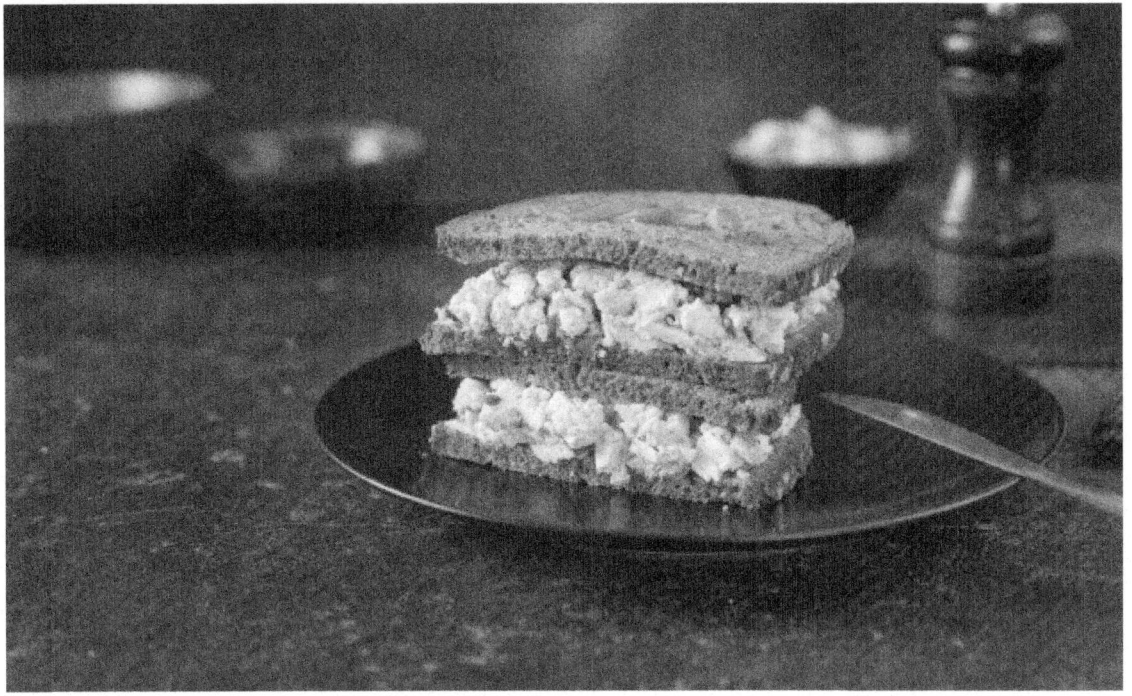

I am sure this is not your first time making egg salad and making sandwiches with it. I used to be petrified when my mom packed some in my lunchbox because they had a distinctive smell. Now, I would do anything to get my mom to make them for me. I make them for my children, and whether they embrace them as they should now, they will later. Here we go.

Serving Size: 2

Cooking Time: 15 Minutes

Ingredients:

- 3 large hardboiled eggs
- 4 slices your favorite bread
- 3 tbsp. mayonnaise
- Salt, pepper
- 1 tbsp. sweet relish
- Pinch smoked paprika.
- Lettuce leaves

Instructions:

1) In a large bowl, mash the cooked eggs with a fork.

2) Add the mayonnaise and all other ingredients.

3) Combine them well and make the texture you prefer. I prefer the texture to be really smooth, some little chunks of eggs.

4) Decide if you want to toast the bread or not and spread the egg mixture generously. Add lettuce if you wish and serve!

A Cobb Salad with Chicken

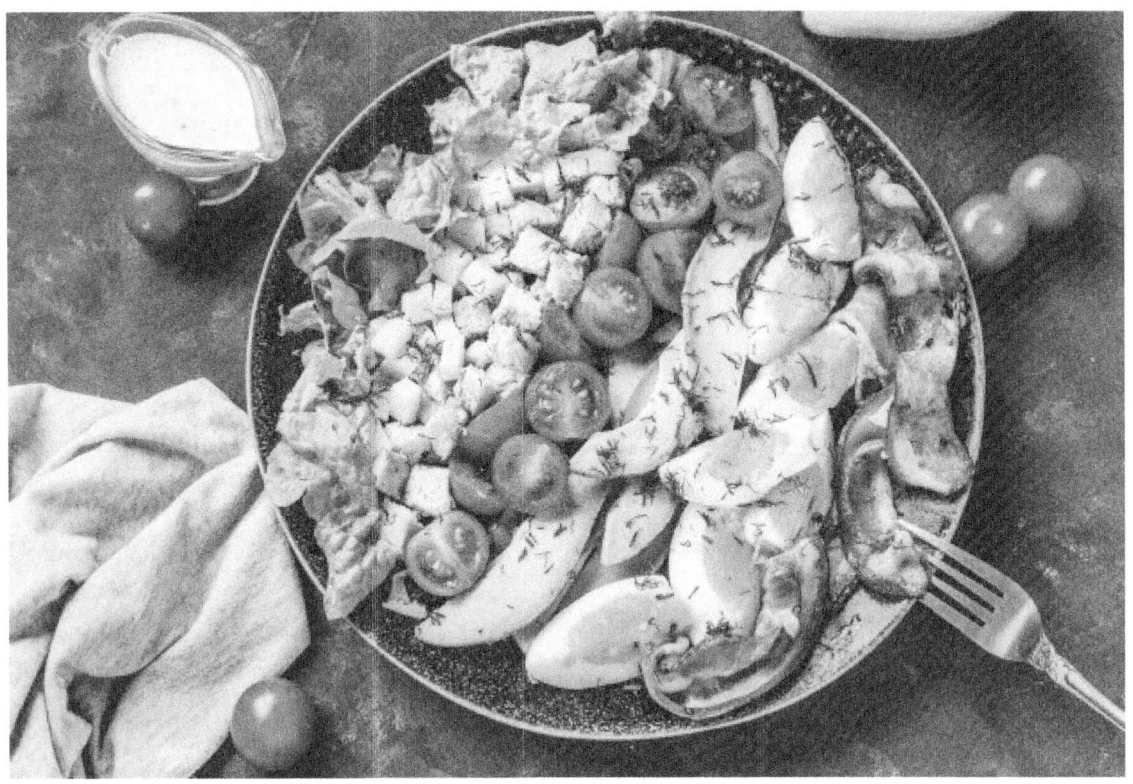

If you order a cobb salad in a restaurant, you will get, for sure, some hardboiled eggs in it. You probably will also get a variety of vegetables, including mixed greens and bacon and ham. This time, we make it a little different and serve it with grilled chicken or even rotisserie chicken, depending on what you have in hand.

Serving Size: 4

Cooking Time: 20 Minutes

Ingredients:

- 4 large hardboiled eggs
- 4 cups mixed greens of your choice
- 12 grape tomatoes
- 1 large avocado, sliced
- 8 slices smoked bacon, cooked to perfection
- 4 cups grilled chicken or rotisserie chicken
- Crumbled blue cheese goat cheese or even shredded American cheese
- 1 minced green onion
- Your favorite salad dressing

Instructions:

1) Get 4 large plates out.

2) Lay a bed of mixed green on each plate and sprinkle the green onion equally.

3) Slice the hardboiled eggs and place them on each bed of lettuce.

4) Also, divide the bacon and chicken equally and the tomatoes.

5) Finally, add the avocado, make the arrangement look pretty. Sprinkle the cheese you chose.

6) Serve with your favorite dressing; I enjoy a chipotle ranch dressing, but choose the one you like.

Fun Eggy Dip

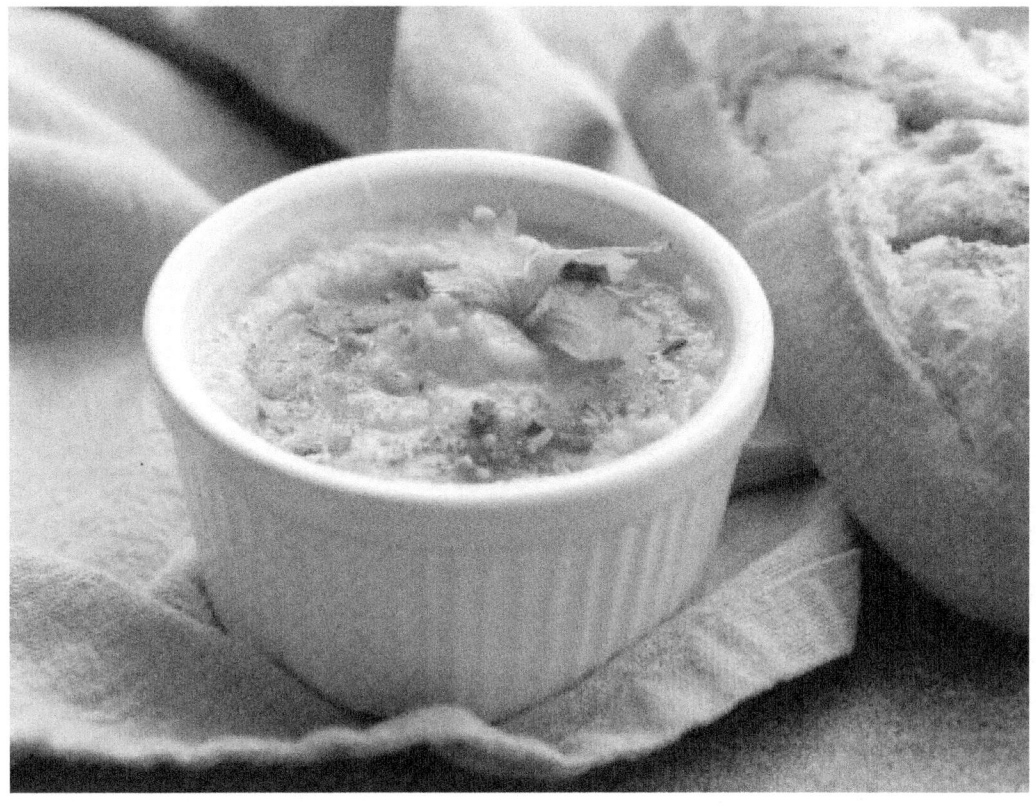

This recipe is easy, and you can add as much as or little spiciness to it. The only rule is to add eggs, make spiciness, and make it wonderful!

Serving Size: 4-8

Cooking Time: 20 Minutes

Ingredients:

- 3 large hardboiled eggs
- 1 cup sour cream
- ½ cup mayonnaise
- 1 tsp. cayenne pepper
- Salt, black pepper
- Minced parsley to decorate.
- Crackers or pita chips

Instructions:

1) Take all the ingredients, except the eggs, and place them in a mixing bowl. Combine.

2) Add the mixture and the hardboiled eggs to the blender.

3) Activate a few times and dump onto a serving bowl. Decorate with minced parsley and serve with your favorite crackers.

Potato Salad with Eggs on top

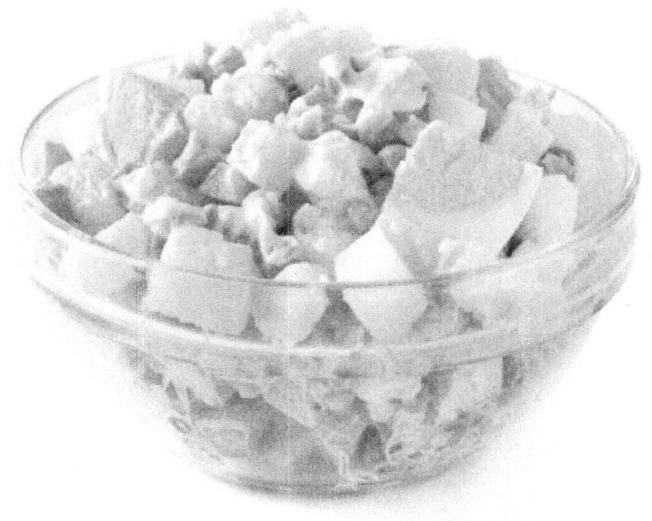

Either you decide to slice hardboiled eggs and incorporate them in potato salad or simply add some on top; you will include them in this recipe. Potato salad can be made in so many ways, and that's what so fabulous about it. When you go to your neighbor's house, your aunt's house, or a work potluck, you will taste so many flavors, although they most likely look just about the same.

Serving Size: 4-6

Cooking Time: 50 Minutes

Ingredients:

- 6 eggs, hardboiled
- 4 large white potatoes
- 1 cup sour cream
- 2 tbsp. mayonnaise
- ½ tbsp. Horseradish sauce
- Salt, black pepper
- 1 tsp. yellow mustard
- Pinch cayenne pepper

Instructions:

1) Get two saucepans out.

2) Bring water and salt to boil in each.

3) In one, you will cook the potatoes you have to previously wash and peel. I suggest to cube them already and cook for about 10 minutes or watch closely; you don't want them to get mushy.

4) The second saucepan is for the hardboiled eggs. You will cook them for 15-20 minutes once the water is boiling; you remove them from the heat.

5) Prepare a large mixing bowl, add the mayonnaise, sour cream, spices, mustard, and Horseradish sauce. Combine well.

6) After the potatoes, the eggs have cooled down and are sliced or cut as you want them, add them carefully into the mixture.

7) Taste and adjust seasonings as needed.

8) There you have your potato salad and keep it in the refrigerator until ready to serve.

Multicolored Macaroni Salad with Eggs

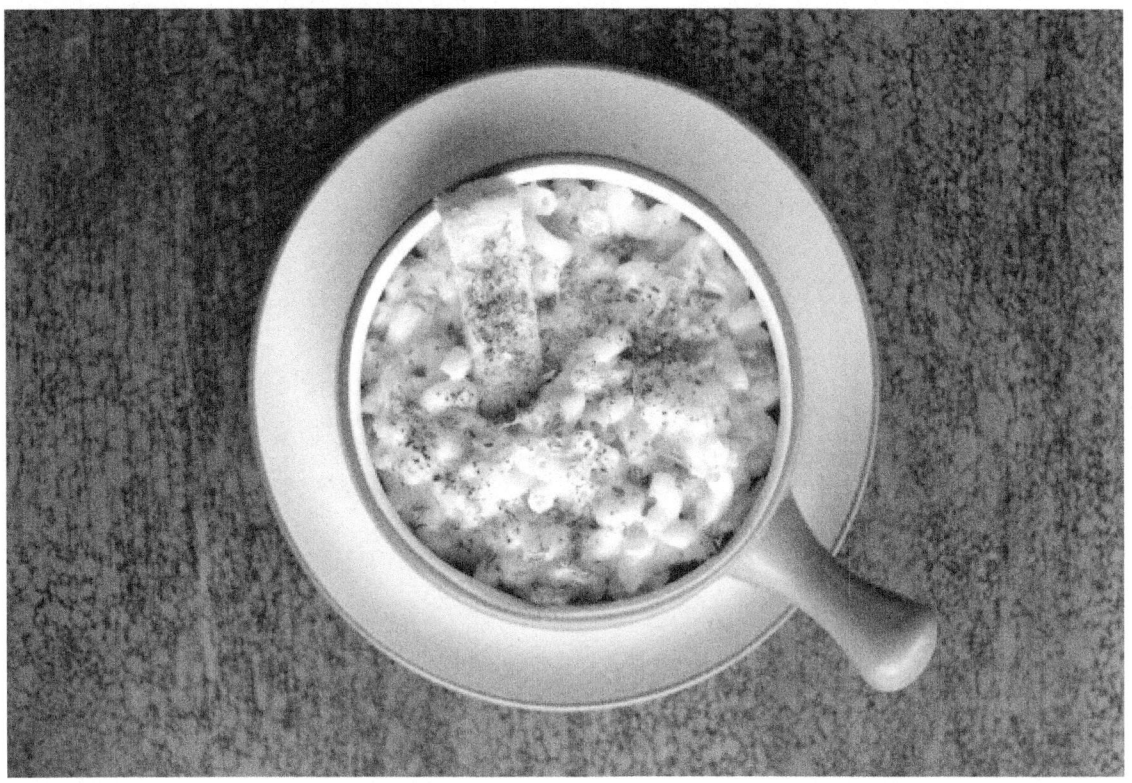

In this salad, the colors will prevail. Oh, wait a minute, the taste also does. We will add ingredients that marry well together but did emphasize choosing several colors. Why choose only white onions when you can select red or green ones? But this time, do not forget eggs!

Serving Size: 4

Cooking Time: 30 Minutes

Ingredients:

- 1 box uncooked macaroni elbow
- ¼ cup diced red onion
- 1 tbsp. minced parsley
- 4 large hardboiled eggs, sliced
- ½ diced yellow bell pepper
- 2 tbsp. Italian dressing
- ½ tsp. minced garlic
- 1.2 cups sour cream
- Salt, black pepper

Instructions:

1) Boil water and salt to cook the pasta and get all the other ingredients out and ready.

2) In a large bowl, combine the sour cream, dressing, and all seasonings.

3) Add the diced onion, minced garlic, and pepper.

4) Once the pasta is done, drain well. Then, let it cool down.

5) Add to the existing mixture and combine well.

6) Finally, add the fresh parsley and sliced hardboiled eggs and keep some parsley for when serving to decorate with.

7) Keep refrigerated when not used.

Breakfast Idea on Pizza

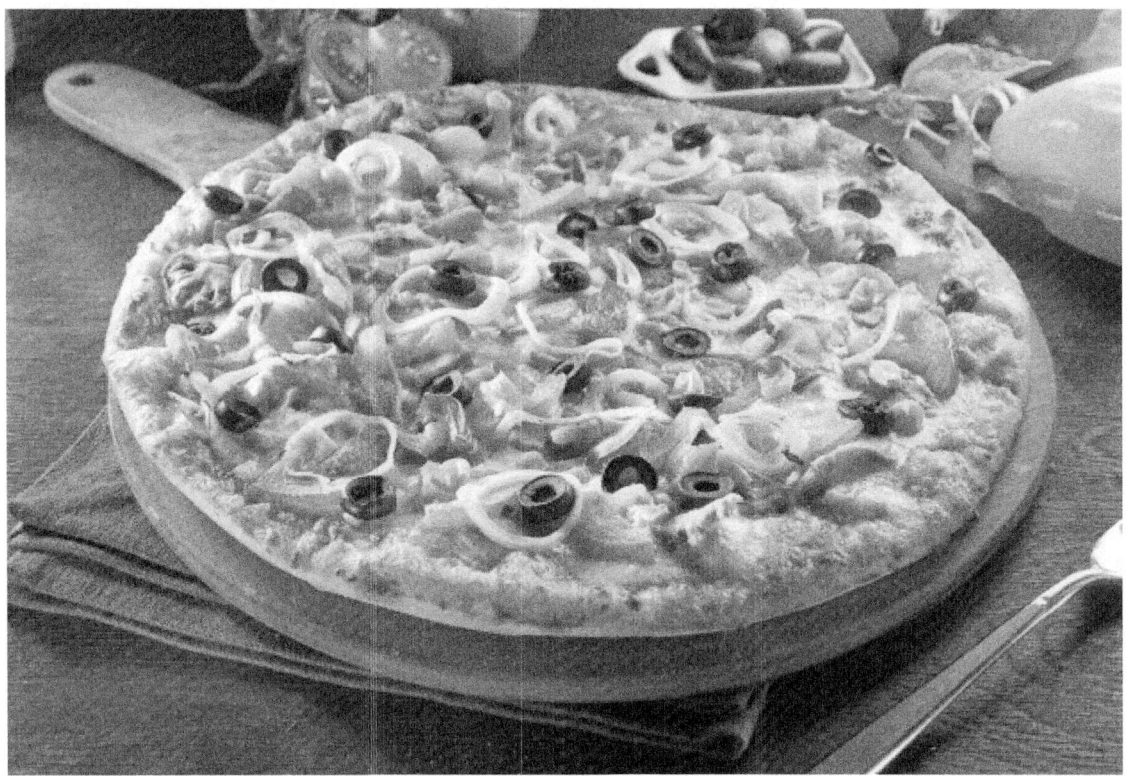

If you cannot get enough breakfast food, this may be a great idea for you. I am one of the people who can make pancakes or eggs and bacon at night and be totally satisfied. Breakfast on a pizza also seems like the perfect solution to satisfy breakfast cravings while giving my family a more dinner like dish.

Serving Size: 3-4

Cooking Time: 40 Minutes

Ingredients:

- 1 large pizza crust
- 1/2 cup crumbled bacon
- ¼ diced red bell pepper
- ½ cup pizza sauce
- 3 medium eggs
- 1 tbsp. whole milk
- Salt, black pepper
- 1 cup shredded Mozzarella cheese
- Some unsalted butter

Instructions:

1) Preheat the oven to 400 degrees F.

2) Next, place the pizza dough on a greased pizza sheet and set it aside.

3) In a small pan, heat some butter.

4) Next, in a mixing bowl, whisk the eggs, milk, salt, and pepper. Cook them into the pan as scrambled eggs.

5) Meanwhile, brush the pizza sauce on the pizza crust, add the bacon, pepper, and scrambled eggs.

6) Then, cover with shredded cheese and place in the oven.

7) Cook for 20-25 minutes or until the cheese has melted and turns golden.

8) Remove and serve hot!

Deviled Eggs Not So Ordinary

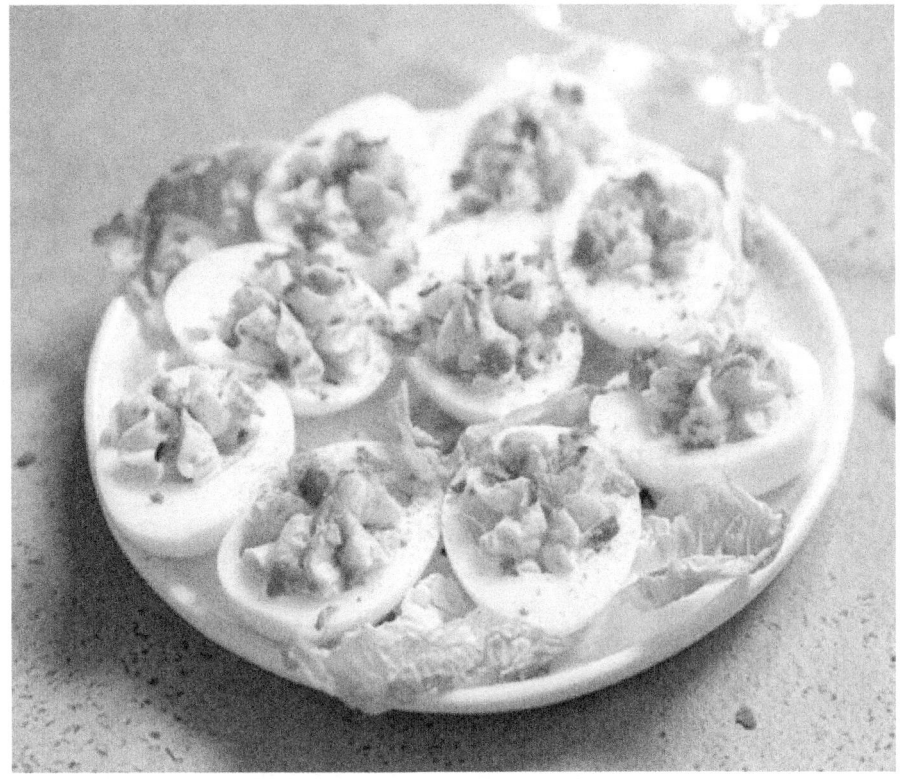

Deviled eggs are devil eggs, many will say. But I do not think it's necessarily true. We can prepare them in so many ways; they can be such a new discovery each time you bite into one. This time, for sure, we will use some hardboiled eggs cut in half, but what matters, where you can let your creativity loose for filling. That is just what we did.

Serving Size: 12

Cooking Time: 60 Minutes

Ingredients:

- 12 large eggs
- ¾ cup mayonnaise
- 1 large can drained white tuna
- 1 tbsp. capers
- ½ tsp. lemon juice
- Salt, black pepper
- ½ tsp. cumin

Instructions:

1) First, boil water in a large saucepan with a little salt. Add the eggs from the beginning, and once the water boils, remove from the heat.

2) Let the eggs cook for 20 minutes.

3) Meanwhile, drain the tuns and add in a large mixing bowl.

4) Next, add the mayonnaise, lemon juice, seasonings, and cappers. Place in the refrigerator for now.

5) When the eggs are done, rinse under cold water and remove the shells.

6) Let them cool them completed before cutting lengthwise.

7) Then, remove the yolks and add them to the mixture you created.

8) Combine and add some more mayonnaise as needed.

9) Stuff all the eggs with this mixture and serve very cold.

Delicious and Simple Angel Hair Pasta with Eggs and more

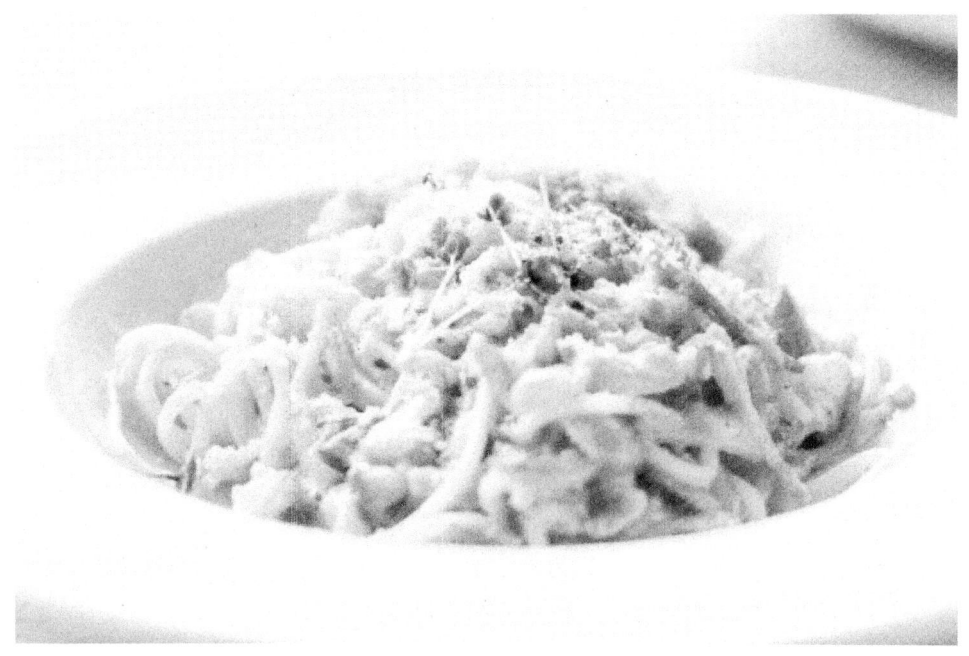

I like fried rice for many reasons, but one of them is because it contains fried eggs. I decided to reciprocate somewhat the same idea but with angel hair pasta. You can or cannot add proteins, such as ham, bacon, or even pork, and make it a complete dish or just serve it as a side dish as you would like.

Serving Size: 4

Cooking Time: 45 Minutes

Ingredients:

- 1 box angel hair pasta
- ½ cup sweet peas
- ¼ cup diced red onion
- 4 large eggs
- Cooking oil
- Salt, black pepper
- 2 tbsp. soy sauce
- Black pepper, salt

Instructions:

1) Cook the pasta in boiling water as you normally do. Remember, angel hair pasta cook fast.

2) Meanwhile, in a large pan, heat the butter and cook the diced onions for 5 minutes.

3) Add the eggs and season with salt, pepper. Scramble it all together and cook.

4) Your pasta should be ready, and drain them well.

5) Add them to the pan, add the sauce and sweet peas and mix all well together.

6) Keep it warm until you are ready to serve.

Egg Benedict in our Way

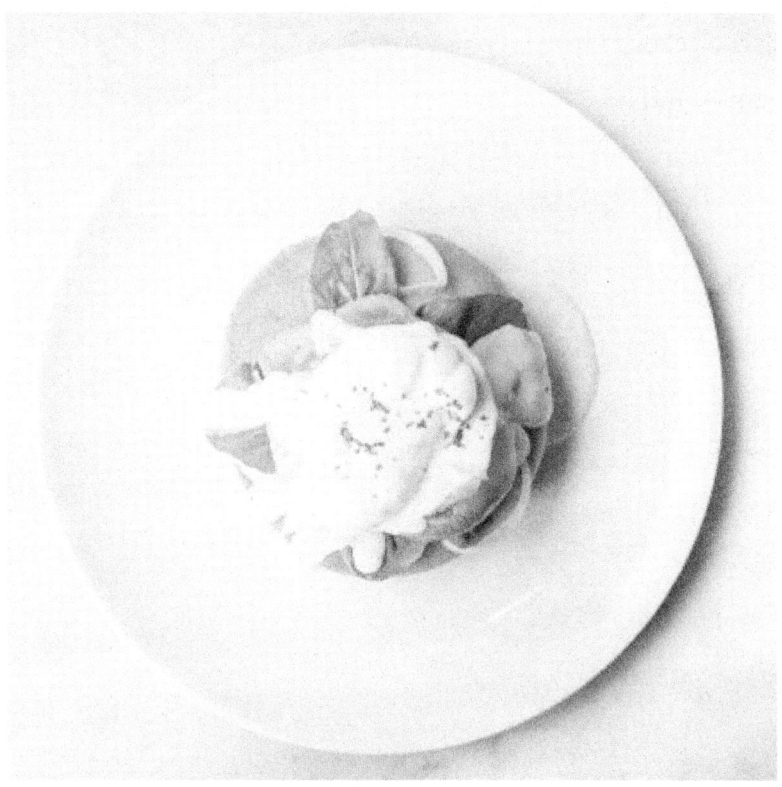

We love to introduce classics in our cookbooks. We also love to twist the classic recipes a little to create our own. We will not compromise Hollandaise sauce; it is a vital ingredient in this egg benedict, and it would not be the same without it. However, a few components will differ, creating a magical new combination of flavors to it. Give it a chance!

Serving Size: 4

Cooking Time: 40 Minutes

Ingredients:

- 4 large eggs
- 4 thick slices cooked ham
- 1 tbsp. whole milk
- 1/tsp. hot sauce
- 4 English muffins (halves) or 2 whole
- Salt, pepper
- Hollandaise sauce
- 3 egg yolks
- ½ tbsp. Dijon mustard
- ½ tbsp. lemon juice
- Pinch salt
- Pinch cayenne pepper
- ½ cup unsalted butter

Instructions:

1) Not only we decided to switch up the poached eggs with scrambled eggs, but we also decided to add a little spiciness to them.

2) You will start by preparing the hollandaise sauce.

3) Melt the butter in a medium saucepan. Add the lemon juice, mustard, seasonings. Make sure all has melted.

4) Get the blender out and dump the mixture into it and add the yolks.

5) Meanwhile, you can scramble your eggs. Then, in a medium bowl, combine the eggs, milk, hot sauce and salt, pepper. Cook them perfectly.

6) Toast the English muffins. Then, place them on the plate. Assemble with a slice of ham, the egg, and a generous portion of hollandaise sauce.

Eggs, Cheese and Ham on Sourdough

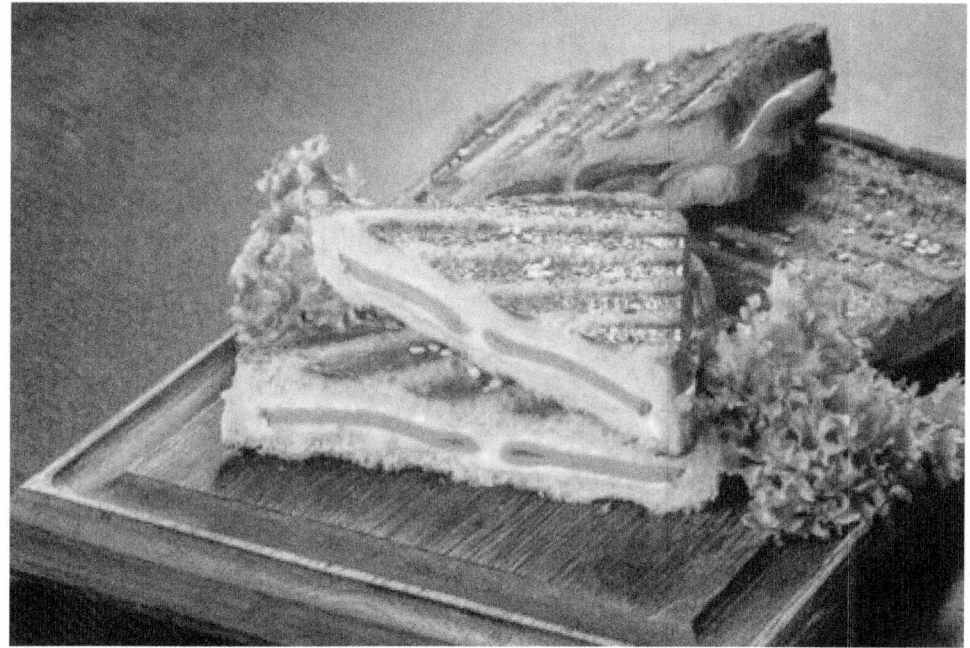

This simple sandwich can go a long way. I think the key ingredient here is the bread you choose. We propose sourdough bread; it has a distinct flavor and density perfect for the occasion. However, you could very well decide to use a whole grain or even baguette to make a sandwich reflecting more your tastes.

Serving Size: 2

Cooking Time: 15 Minutes

Ingredients:

- 4 slices deli smoked ham
- 4 slices sourdough bread or any bread you picked
- 2 large eggs
- Salt, black pepper
- Little butter

Instructions:

1) This is an easy and delicious breakfast.

2) Melt a little butter in a pan and cook the eggs sunny side up.

3) Toast the bread and spread butter on each piece.

4) Assemble with the eggs in the middle and a slice of ham on each side.

5) Enjoy with a coffee or orange juice.

Weekend Potato and Egg Casserole

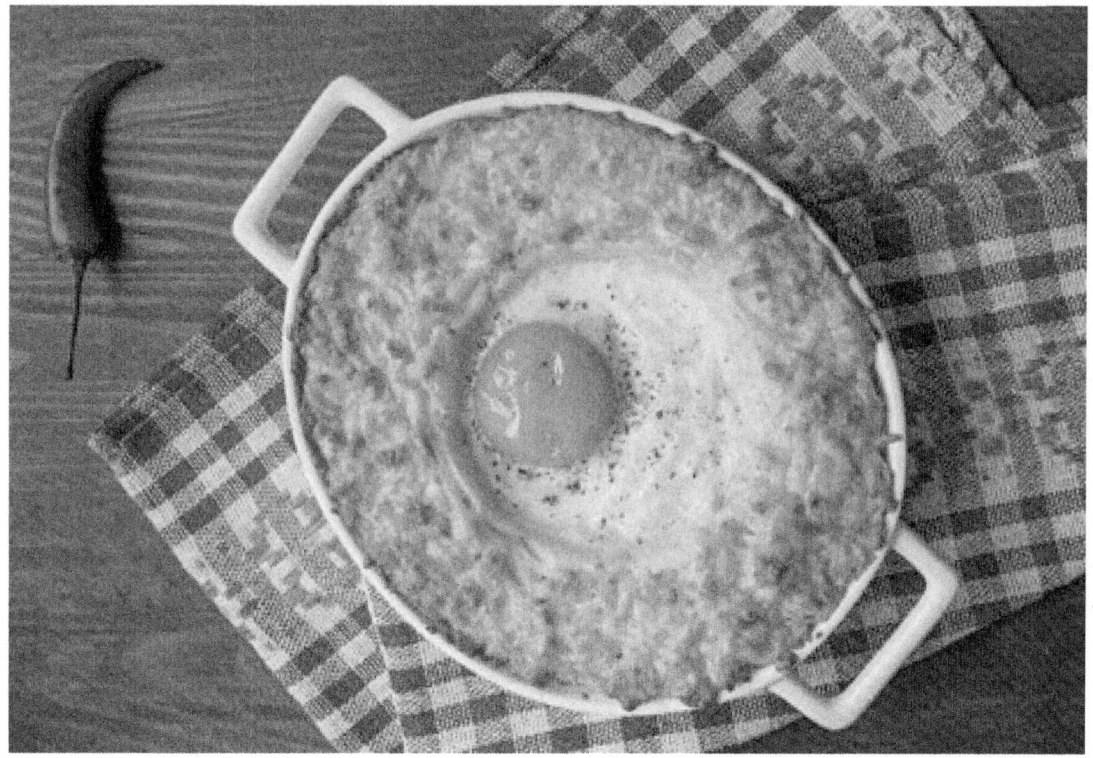

I love waking up to the smell of breakfast food. I have to say it does not happen as I am the main cook in the household after all! So, I pay forward and prepare breakfast on weekends, hoping my children will reciprocate one day or pass on the tradition to their own children. This potato casserole is a tricky way to add some veggies to their breakfast.

Serving Size: 4

Cooking Time: 40 Minutes

Ingredients:

- 2 large diced red skin potatoes
- 2 large diced sweet potatoes
- 4 large eggs
- ½ diced sweet onion
- 1 tbsp. minced garlic
- 1 tbsp. fresh minced rosemary
- Unsalted butter

Instructions:

1) This is when I really appreciate the microwave to give me a head start. I wash and place the potatoes into a microwave friendly dish.

2) I usually cook two potatoes at a time for about 7 minutes.

3) Remove them and diced them as they have softened some.

4) Gather all the ingredients and start cooking.

5) Melt some butter in a large skillet and add the onions and garlic. Cook for 5 minutes.

6) Add all the diced potatoes and season them and also add the fresh rosemary. Stir often. They should be cooked for about 20 minutes.

7) Five minutes before potatoes are ready. Grab another pan and heat butter. Cook the 4 eggs sunny side up and serve them on a hot bed of potatoes.

Baked Potatoes with Chives, Bacon and Eggs

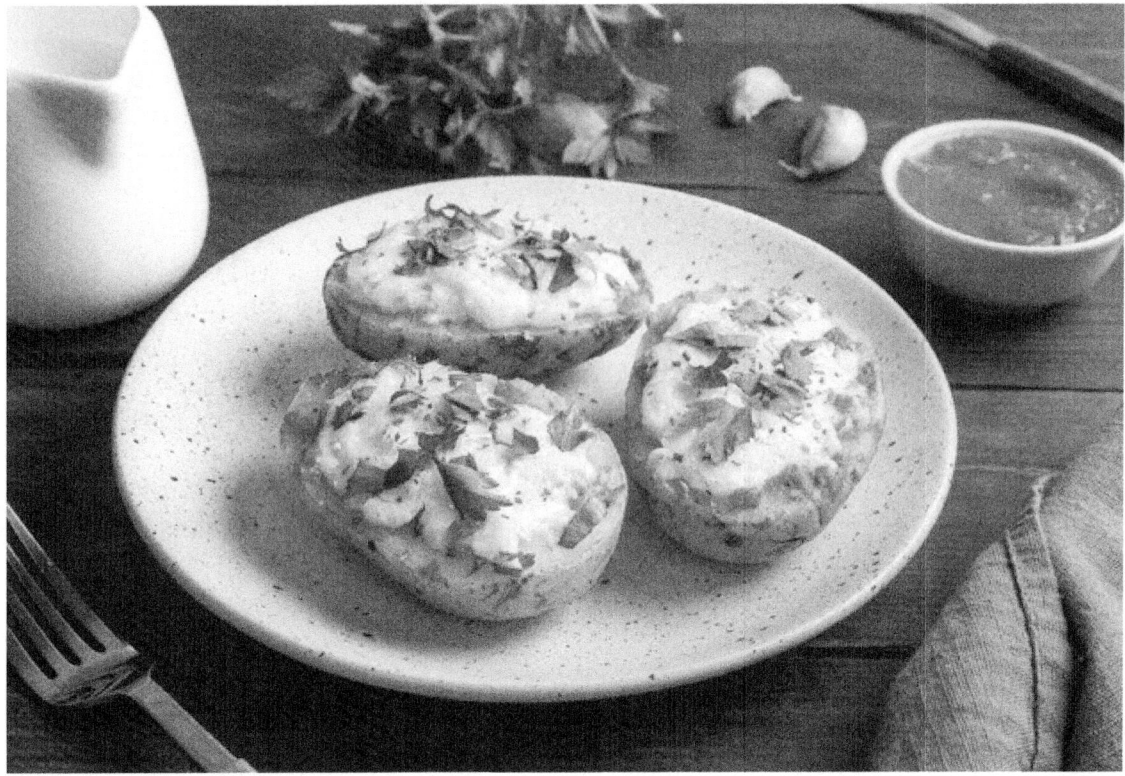

I was earlier talking about how fun and delicious it can be to stuff vegetables with an egg mixture. Here is another great idea. Using potatoes allows you to cook this breakfast slowly. It is not the recipe to choose if you are in a hurry in the morning. I prefer greatly to bake them as opposed to use the microwave for cooking them. For sure, you can pre-cook them, but the flavors of baked potatoes don't equal the flavors of microwaved ones.

Serving Size: 4

Cooking Time: 60 Minutes

Ingredients:

- 4 large golden potatoes
- 4 crumbled pieces bacon
- 1 cup shredded sharp Cheddar
- 4 large eggs
- Salt and black pepper
- 2 tbsp. cream
- 1 tbsp. minced fresh chives
- Sour cream
- Unsalted butter

Instructions:

1) First, preheat the oven to 400 degrees F.

2) Wash the potatoes and 2 at a time, precook in the microwave for about 5 minutes.

3) Cut lengthwise and remove the flesh – if they are not soft enough, cook for another minute at a time in the microwave.

4) Next, whisk the eggs and cream with salt and pepper in a large mixing bowl. Place the potatoes flesh into the bowl.

5) Add the bacon and chives and combine.

6) Place the egg mixture into each potato. Add the cheese on top.

7) Then, place the potatoes into a greased baking dish and bake for another 30 minutes.

8) Serve with sour cream.

Crustless Spinach and Cheese Quiche

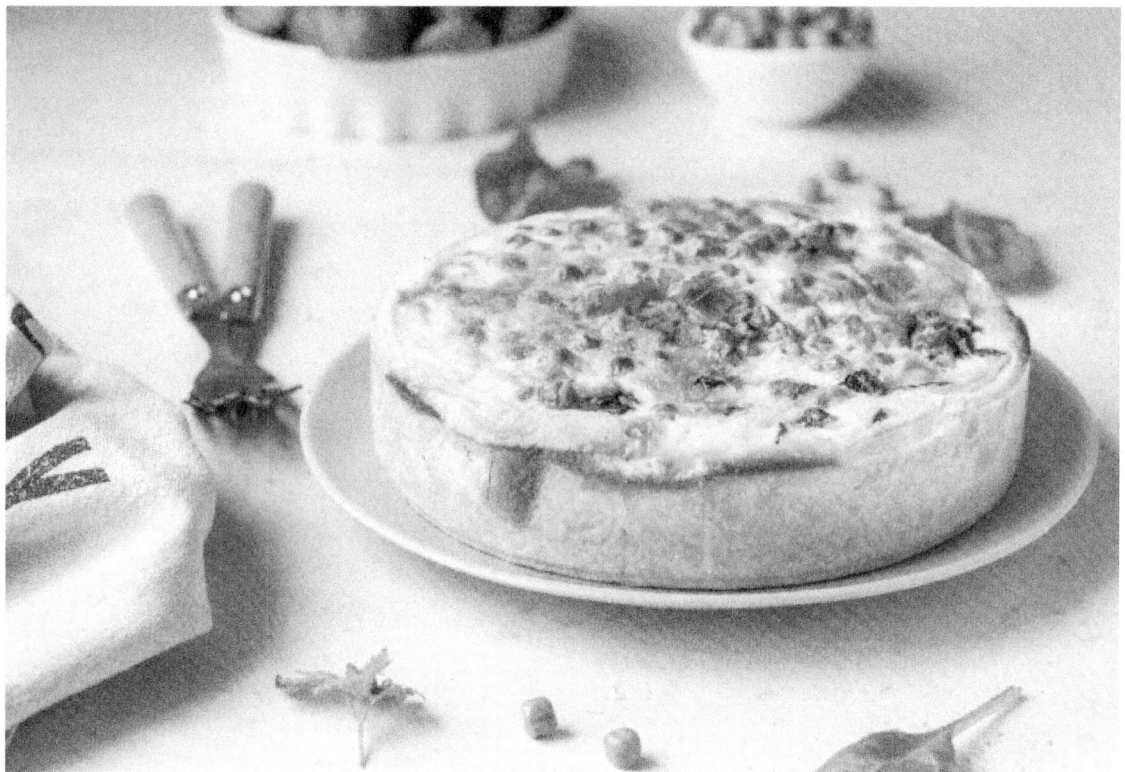

No surprise here. We use eggs in a quiche. The surprise here is that we will prepare a crustless quiche. It will be about the same ingredients but without the crust! Let us make sure the quiche is well done also after baking, so it does not fall apart when serving. Also, it is important that you wait until it has cool down a little before sling; if not, it will definitely crumble, and you will not be left with a pretty slice of it to serve.

Serving Size: 4

Cooking Time: 60 Minutes

Ingredients:

- 6 large eggs
- 2 cups prewashed baby spinach leaves
- 1 small sliced zucchini
- ¼ cup diced sweet onion
- ½ tbsp. minced garlic
- 1 cup shredded Mozzarella cheese
- 1 cup cottage cheese
- Unsalted butter
- Salt, black pepper
- Pinch ground cumin
- Pinch ground nutmeg

Instructions:

1) Preheat the oven to 375 degrees f.

2) Spray with oil a pie pan. Set aside.

3) In a large pan, heat some butter and add the onion, garlic, and zucchini. Cook for 5-6 minutes. Then, add the spinach, season with salt and pepper, and cook for another 2 minutes. Set aside.

4) In a large mixing bowl, whisk the eggs. Add the cottage cheese and cooked veggies. Combine.

5) Finally, add the mozzarella cheese, the seasonings and combine once more.

6) Dump this mixture into the pie pan.

7) Bake in the oven for 45-50 minutes.

8) Serve with hot sauce if you like.

Omelet Loaded with Meat and Love

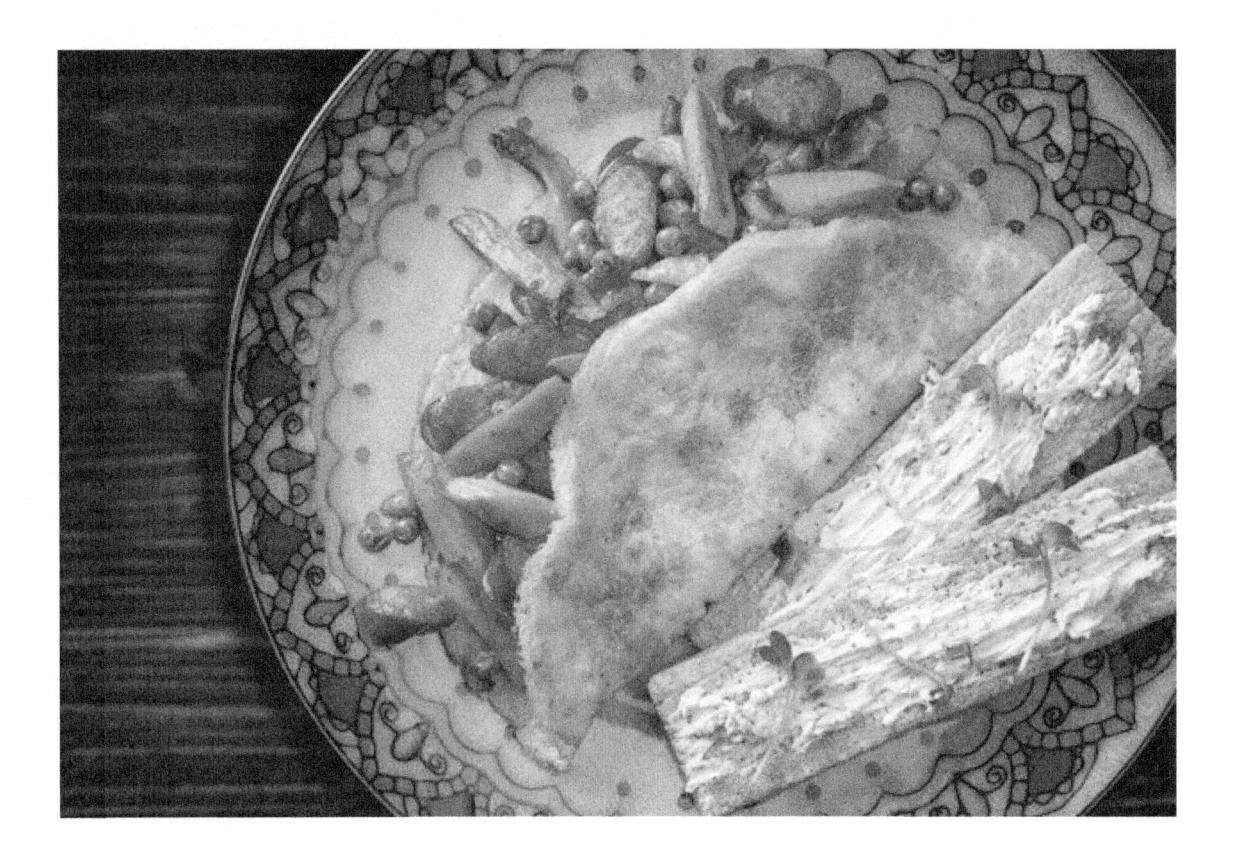

This omelet is made for meat lovers. If you are the type who orders pizza with the most meats on top, then you will love it. This is a great option when you have leftover ham, bacon, sausages, or pepperoni. I think any of the meats is fair game, depending on your taste. We will give you suggestions below and make it your own, as always!

Serving Size: 4

Cooking Time: 45 Minutes

Ingredients:

- 1 tbsp. fresh cream
- 4 large eggs
- ½ cup diced pepperoni
- ½ cup diced cooked ham
- ½ cup cooked Italian sausage
- 1 cup shredded Swiss cheese
- Salt, black pepper
- Some unsalted butter

Instructions:

1) Gather all ingredients and a medium pan.

2) Whish the eggs, cream and salt, pepper.

3) One at a time, add a quarter of the mixture in the hot pan.

4) Cook the omelet as you would normally knowing that you will fold it soon. Do not overcook.

5) While still flat, add a portion of meat and cheese in the omelet and fold.

6) Cook another few minutes on each side to let the cheese melt and the meats warm up.

7) Serve while it is hot! Repeat the same procedure for the other omelets.

Eggs in a Creamy Bechamel Sauce

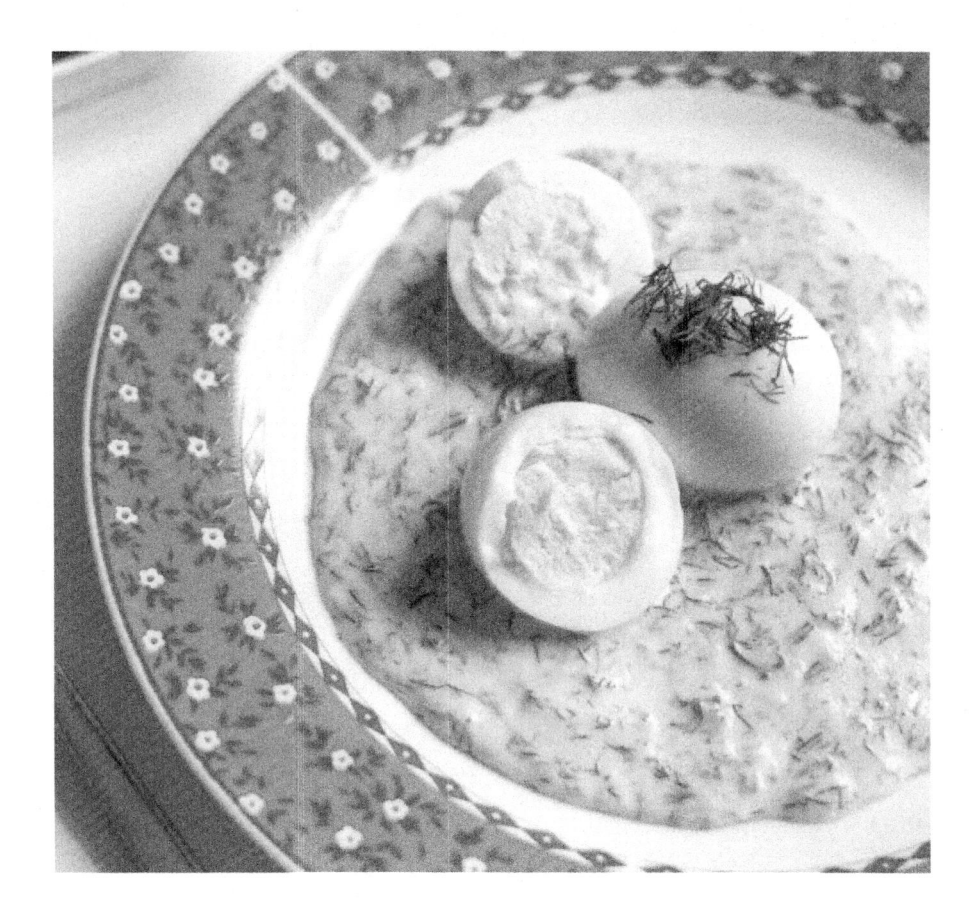

This is a dish that is dear to me. It does remind me of my mother. My mother is French, and she loved to see bechamel sauce on many proteins. The eggs with the white sauce, we called it as we were kids. We ask for the dish over and over. Now, I am sharing with you because sharing is caring. Serve it with a side of green veggies to make a statement.

Serving Size: 4

Cooking Time: 40 Minutes

Ingredients:

- 4 large hardboiled eggs
- Green veggies you choose
- 4 toasts
- Bechamel sauce
- 2 tbsp. unsalted butter
- 1 tbsp. cornstarch
- 1 tbsp. all-purpose flour
- Pinch salt
- 1 1/14 cups whole milk (hot)
- Black pepper
- Pinch nutmeg

Instructions:

1) To make the sauce, you will use a medium saucepan. Melt the butter and add the flour and cornstarch. Keep stirring constantly.

2) It will become pasty. Do not let it get dark.

3) Next, add the hot milk and continue stirring. The sauce will thicken.

4) Add the salt, pepper, and nutmeg. Stir and keep it on low heat.

5) Then, slice the hardboiled eggs and place them on a piece of bread you just toasted.

6) Add a generous portion of bechamel sauce.

7) Lastly, serve with a side of your favorite green veggies.

Eggs on a Baguette

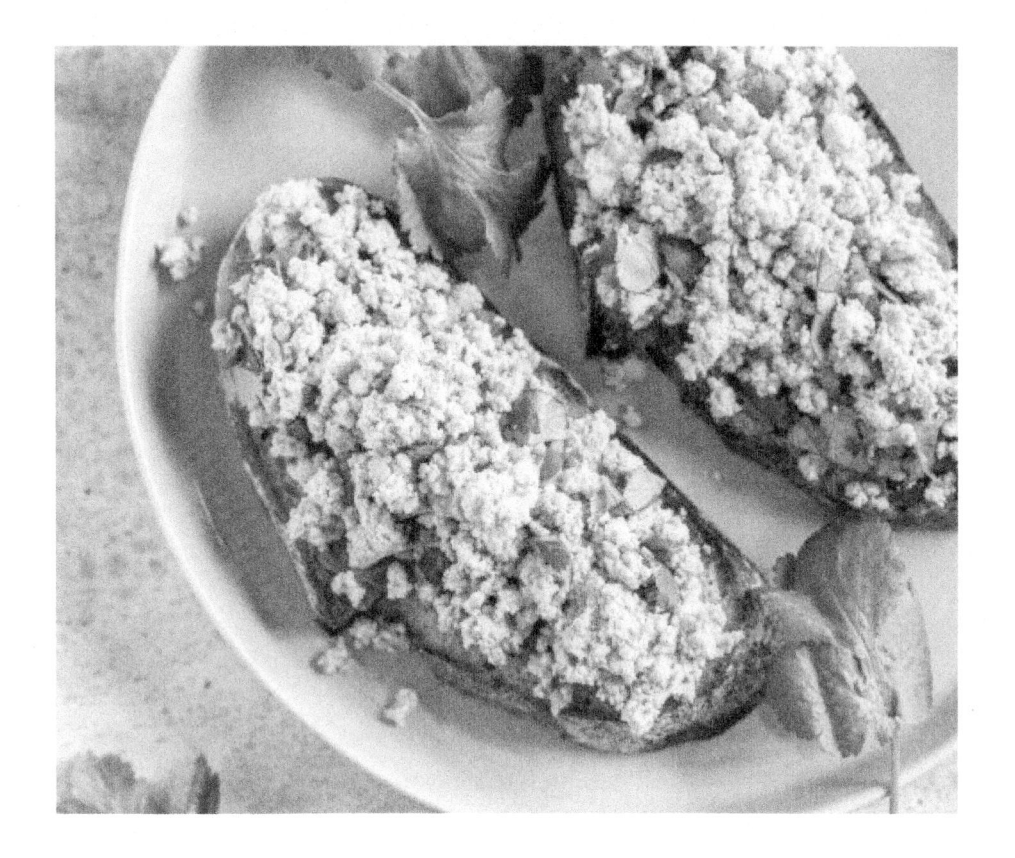

I think it is difficult to go wrong with baguettes. They are crispy, fresh, and simply delicious. It is a celebration at home when I come back from the bakery with a baguette. It is a surprise for everyone when I wake up extra early to go get it first thing in the morning and call out that I am making eggs on a baguette. Get creative and add what you love to the scrambled egg mixture.

Serving Size: 2-3

Cooking Time: 30 Minutes

Ingredients:

- 1 large baguette
- 4 large eggs
- 1 minced green onion
- Unsalted butter
- 1 tbsp. whole milk
- ¾ cup shredded Parmesan cheese

Instructions:

1) Preheat the oven to 400 degrees F.

2) In a pan, melt the butter while whisking the eggs, salt, pepper, and milk in a bowl.

3) Add the egg mixture into the pan and cook the scrambled eggs lightly.

4) Cut the baguette in lengthwise and then again in half, so you have 4 pieces.

5) Place the scrambled eggs on top and then the Parmesan cheese.

6) Bake in the oven for 15 minutes and serve.

Breakfast or Lunch Egg and Veggie Quesadillas

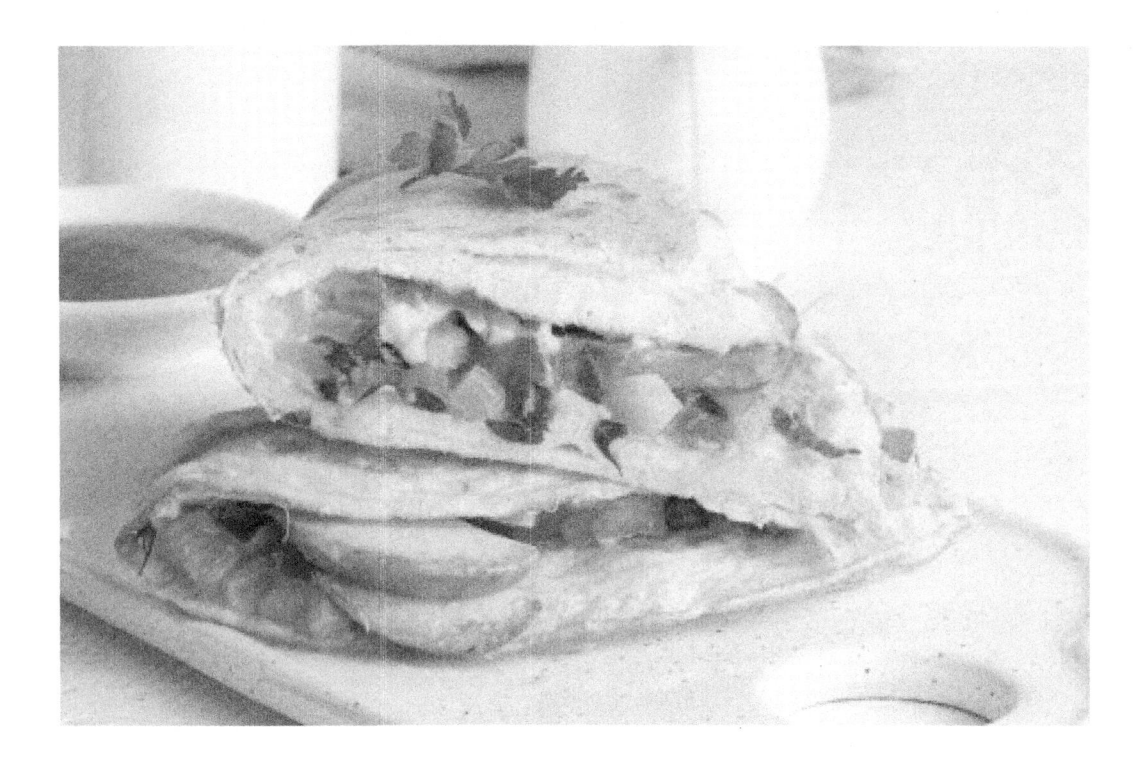

Breakfast is not only a breakfast meal, but it can also be eaten at any meal of the day. Quesadillas are not only a dinner item, but they can also be eaten at any time of the day. For that reason, we are combining eggs and quesadillas and choosing the middle meal of the day, a lunch. Just because I have some spiciness lovers at home, so I typically add a hot sauce in my egg mixture or simply put a bottle of it on the table for them to enjoy.

Serving Size: 2

Cooking Time: 20 Minutes

Ingredients:

- 2 medium tortilla breads
- 1 cup fresh baby spinach
- ½ tsp. garlic powder
- Salt, black pepper
- ½ cup crumbled feta cheese
- 2 large eggs
- 1 tbsp. whole milk
- Unsalted butter

Instructions:

1) Cook the eggs first. Mix the eggs with milk and salt, pepper in a medium bowl.

2) Heat butter in a pan and cook scrambled eggs. Set aside.

3) Add a little butter and cook the spinach for just a few minutes with garlic powder. Set aside.

4) Clean the pan. Heat a little more butter.

5) Lay the tortilla breads and fill them with eggs and spinach. Add crumbled Feta cheese and fold.

6) Cook in the pan on each side for about 3-4 minutes.

7) Serve right away.

The Egg Drop Soup, just a little Different.

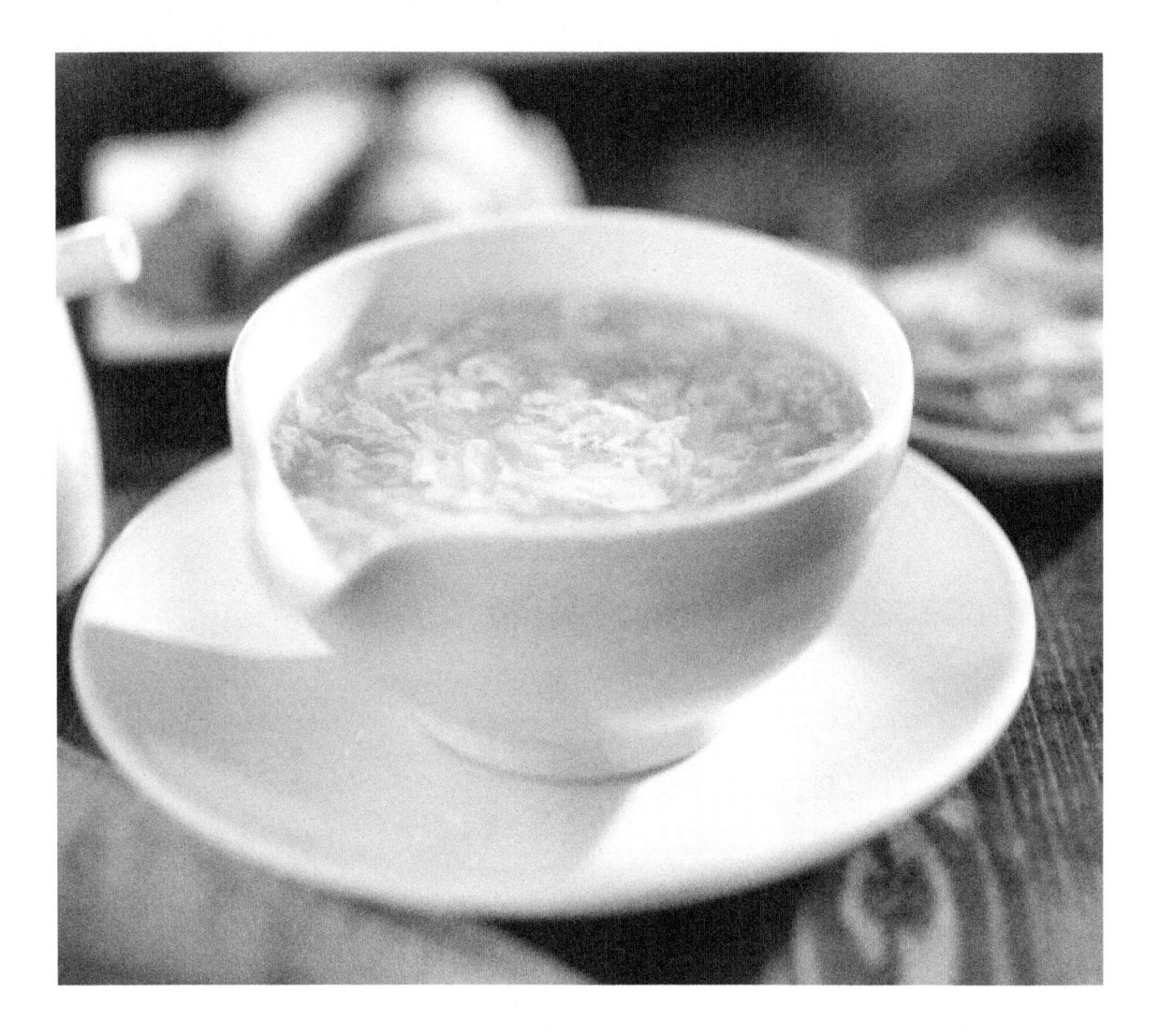

What a staple at any Chinese or Japanese restaurant to offer an egg drop soup on their menu. I have been making the type of soup at a young age, without even knowing it. We used to cook many fondues at home, and with the leftover bouillon, the next day, we would heat it and crack eggs in it, making a delicious salty and satisfying soup. This soup here is different, and, of course, we will not ask you to cook a fondue first. But it will be equally delicious.

Serving Size: 4-6

Cooking Time: 40 Minutes

Ingredients:

- 6 cups chicken broth
- ½ envelop onion soup mix
- 1 tbsp. soy sauce
- 4-5 large eggs
- 1 tbsp. white balsamic vinegar
- Pinch black pepper
- 1 minced green onion

Instructions:

1) Get a large saucepan out.

2) Combine in it the broth, seasonings, sauce, vinegar and onion soup mix.

3) Let it simmer for at least 15 minutes.

4) Few minutes before eating, bring to boil.

5) Crack the eggs into the soup and stir, so they become stringy.

6) When the eggs are cooked, divide the soup into 4 bowls.

7) Add minced green onions on top.

Breakfast Burritos Better than at the Restaurant

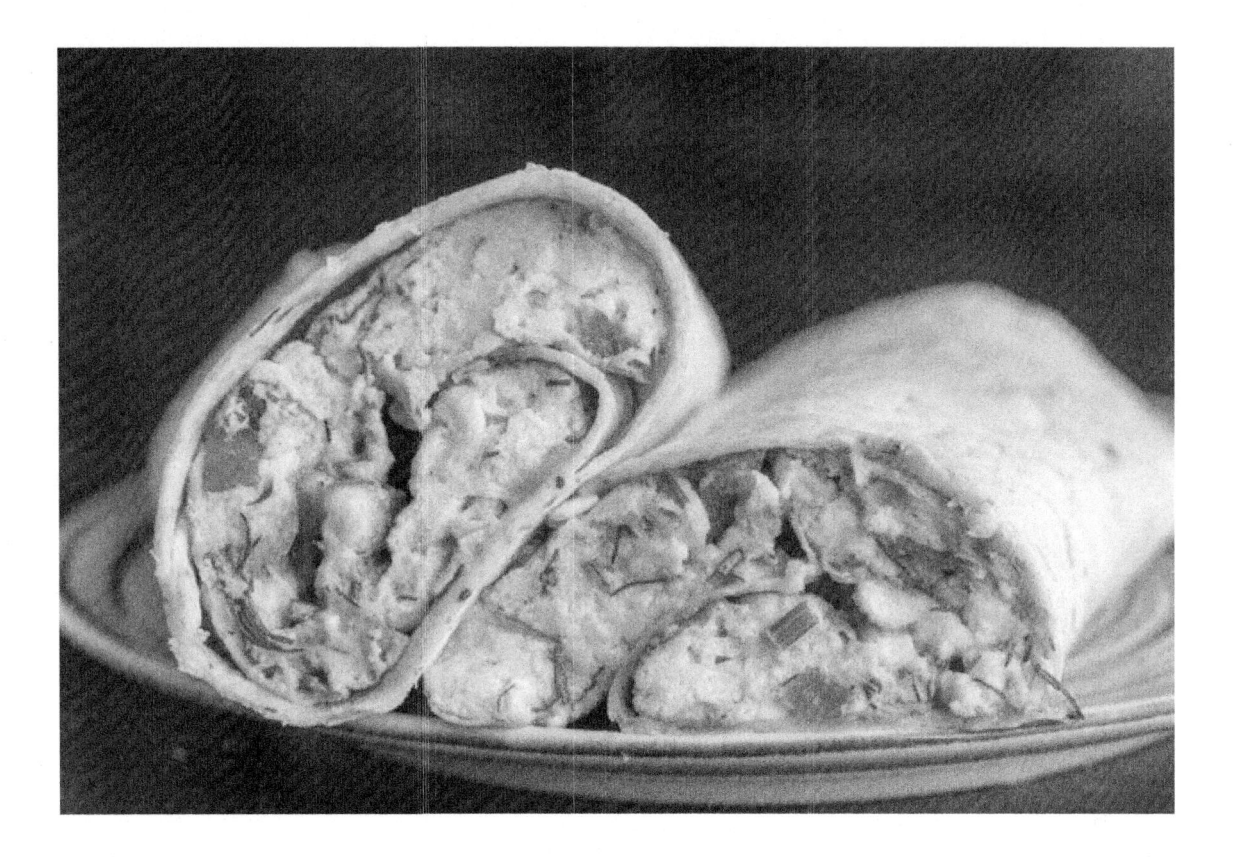

Why would these be better? Because they are homemade, first of all. Because you can add exactly what you want and love in each of them. Because they will invade your home with the richness of their smell when cooking them. Are they enough reasons? How about you can sneak some vegetables in them if your little ones are not a big fan of vegetables? Also, you can make the breakfast meal any time of the day, because your loved ones simply will not mind.

Serving Size: 2

Cooking Time: 20 Minutes

Ingredients:

- 2 medium sized white tortilla breads
- ½ diced avocado
- 2 large eggs
- Few drops hot sauce
- 1 tbsp. 2% milk
- Salt, black pepper
- ½ cup diced smoked deli ham
- Unsalted Butter

Instructions:

1) Heat a medium pan and melt a little butter.

2) In a bowl, whisk the eggs, hot sauce, ham, milk and salt, pepper.

3) Cook the eggs, scrambled in the pan.

4) Meanwhile, lay flat the tortillas, add diced avocados.

5) When the eggs are ready, divide them into 2 portions and place them in the tortillas.

6) Roll up the bread to form a burrito.

Eggs, Sausage and a whole lot more Casserole

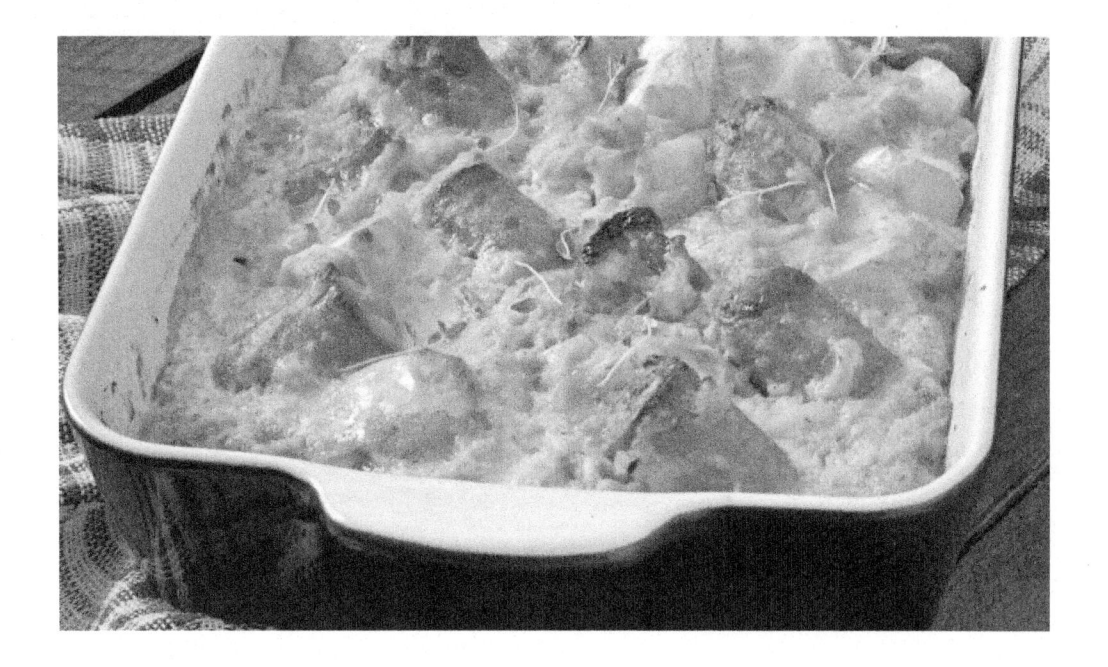

Warm up your oven and get ready to be warmed up on a cold winter day with this lovely recipe. Casseroles have a way to make us feel better no matter what. With the comfort of all of the ingredients mixing perfectly together and the warmth of the dish combined, it will be a success every time. What I love about this dish is that you can once again modify it as you please. If you are vegetarian, you can surely make it free of meats.

Serving Size: 4-6

Cooking Time: 50 Minutes

Ingredients:

- 3 cups cooked crumbled breakfast sausages
- 6 large eggs
- 2 cups Ricotta cheese
- ½ cup sour cream
- 1 cup shredded Mozzarella cheese
- ½ diced red bell pepper
- 1/2 diced red onion
- Salt, black pepper
- 1 tbsp. red pepper flakes
- Minced fresh parsley
- Little cooking oil

Instructions:

1) Preheat the oven to 400 degrees F.

2) Grease a large baking dish. Then, set it aside.

3) In a medium pan, heat a little oil and cook the onion and pepper for 5 minutes. Set aside.

4) In a large mixing bowl, whisk the eggs.

5) Add the sour cream and ricotta cheese and seasonings. Combine.

6) Add the cooked veggies and the cooked sausage and combine again.

7) Dump the mixture into the dish and cover with shredded Mozzarella.

8) Bake in the oven for 45 minutes.

9) Serve with salsa if you wish.

Hearty Bacon and Egg Soup

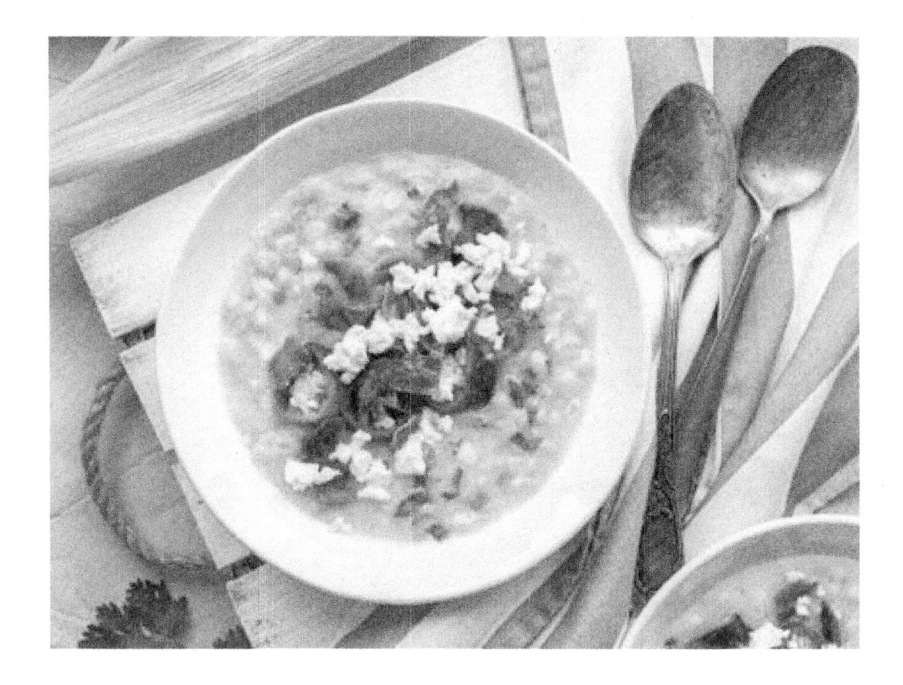

It is time to make another soup with your eggs. We told you we would suggest some recipes outside of the box. Eggs and soup may not normally go together, but we do make them work here. Eggs, bacon, and kale definitely go together in a soup that is definitely appealing. So, we are reuniting the three ingredients and more and making this hearty soup today.

Serving Size: 4

Cooking Time: 50 Minutes

Ingredients:

- 6 cups vegetable broth
- 1 tbsp. dried Italian herbs seasonings
- 6 slices cooked smoked bacon
- 1 large can seasoned red kidney beans or black ones if you prefer
- 2 cups washed and chopped fresh kale
- 1 tbsp. minced garlic
- 1 small chopped yellow onion
- Salt, black pepper
- Unsalted butter
- 4 large eggs

Instructions:

1) Get a large pot out. Melt a little butter and add the garlic and onions. Cook 5 minutes.

2) Add the broth and the salt, pepper, and herbs.

3) Keep on medium heat and add the beans, kale, and bacon. Let the soup simmer for a while, about 30 minutes, so the flavors blend well.

4) 5 minutes before serving. Melt butter in a medium pan and cook all 4 eggs, assuming you are serving 4 people, sunny side up.

5) Portion the soup into 4 bowls and add the cooked egg on top.

6) Dig in!

Fun Breakfast Idea for Children

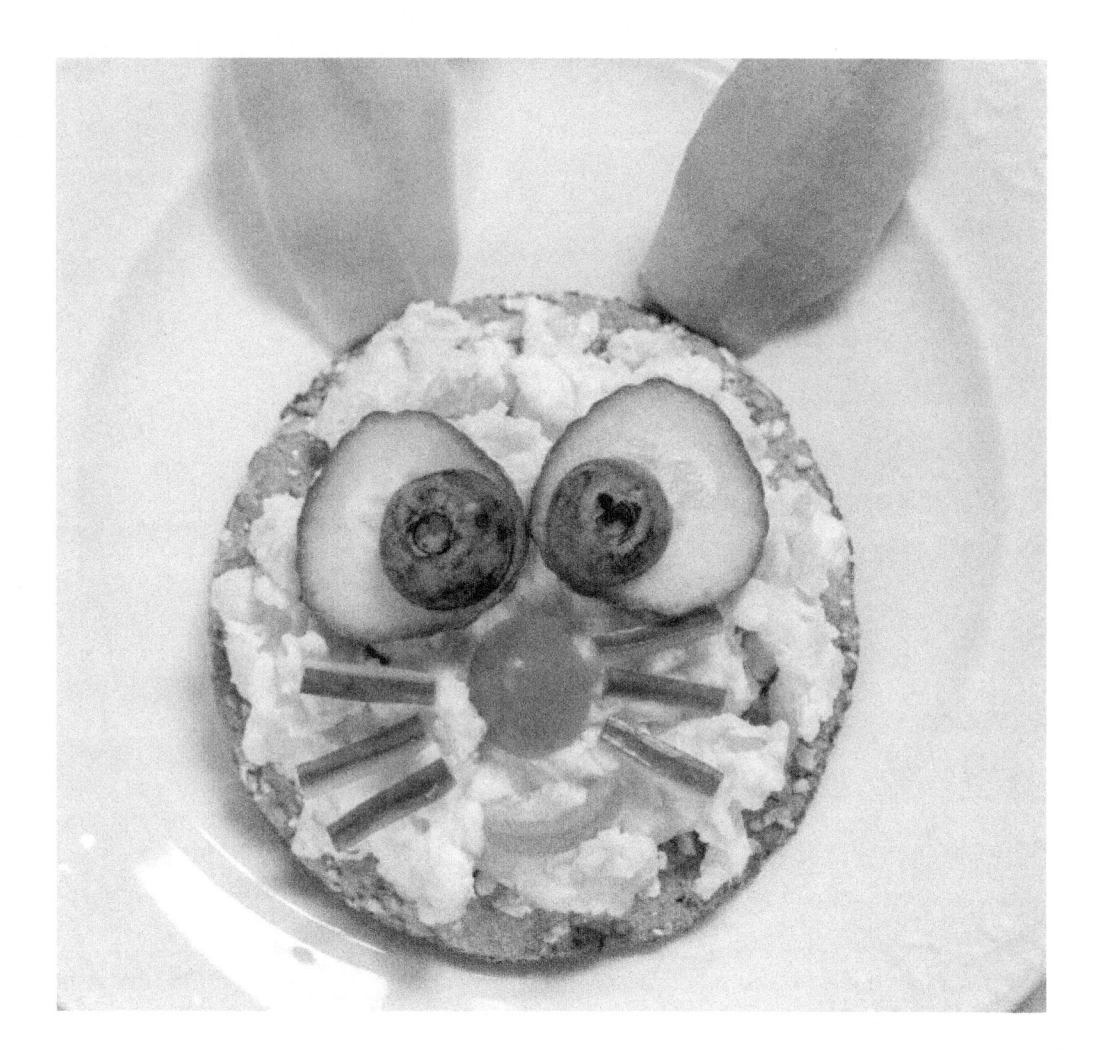

Do you have a toddler who refuses to eat in the mornings? I had one of my children who refused to eat most mornings until I discovered just how to attract them in the kitchen. I decided to involve them in the making of their own breakfast. It was a winning solution. Either you are making smiley face pancakes or creating a smile with ketchup on eggs, the key is to let your children help you and tell what they would like to make. Introduce eggs along the way.

Serving Size: 1

Cooking Time: 20 Minutes

Ingredients:

- 1 large egg
- Pinch salt
- 2 black olives
- 1 cheese stick
- 4 slices pepperoni
- 1 grape tomato
- Salt, black pepper

Instructions:

1) Get a large white plate out.

2) In a small bowl, whisk the egg and season with salt and pepper.

3) Cook the egg, scrambled.

4) Cut the pepperoni in halves, and then again, you have mouth shaped pieces. Also, peel the cheese stick in strings.

5) When the eggs are cooked, place them in the center of the plate. Use the olives for the eyes. The cheese strings for the hair. The pepperoni for the mouth and a grape tomato for the nose! You will have extra pepperoni; you can use them for the ears or a tie, be creative.

Chicken Parmesan and Egg Meet

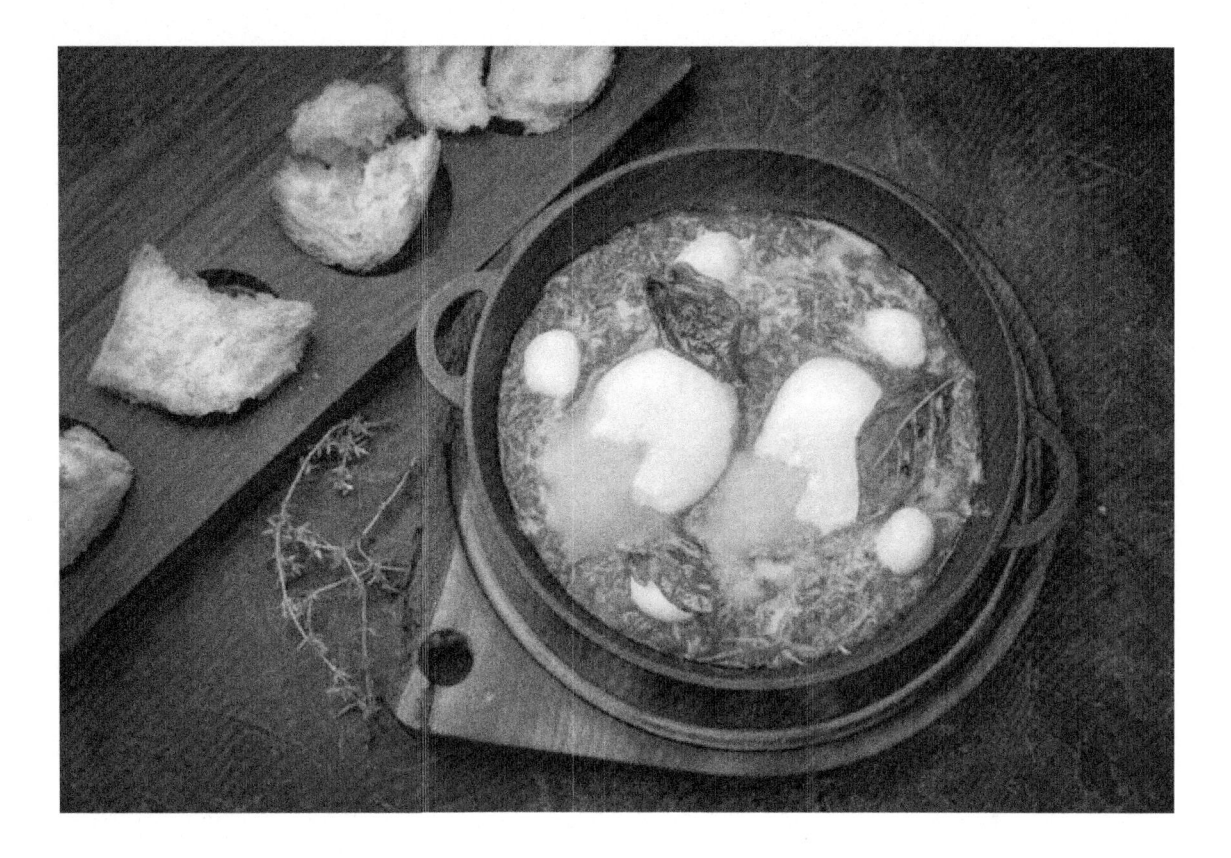

This may not be the breakfast you anticipated. It is surely not one to create when you are in a hurry. You will need your oven unless you already have precooked chicken breasts, as it is time consuming. You can, for sure, consider the dish as a hearty dinner, as it contains proteins and can be a heavy side dish if you are not a breakfast person. You can also surprise your family and do not tell them in advance that you are adding eggs to the traditional dish.

Serving Size: 4

Cooking Time: 60 Minutes

Ingredients:

- 4 boneless and skinless chicken breasts
- 2 cups your favorite spaghetti sauce
- Cooked fettuccine noodles
- 1 cup grated Parmesan cheese
- 4 large eggs
- Salt, pepper
- Unsalted butter

Instructions:

1) Preheat the oven to 375 degrees F.

2) Next, grease a large baking dish and set it aside.

3) Season the chicken breasts on each side and place on the dish. Then, add the sauce on top and the cheese on top of the sauce.

4) Bake as you usually would, about 30-35 minutes. Make sure the chicken is cooked all the way.

5) Meanwhile, get the eggs out and 4 plates.

6) When the chicken is cooked, remove it from the oven. Cook four sunny side up eggs.

7) Then, plate one breast of chicken on each plate on a bed of fettuccine. Add one egg on top and season with salt, pepper.

8) It would be even more enjoyable with a glass of wine!

Beautiful and Delicious Breakfast Avocados

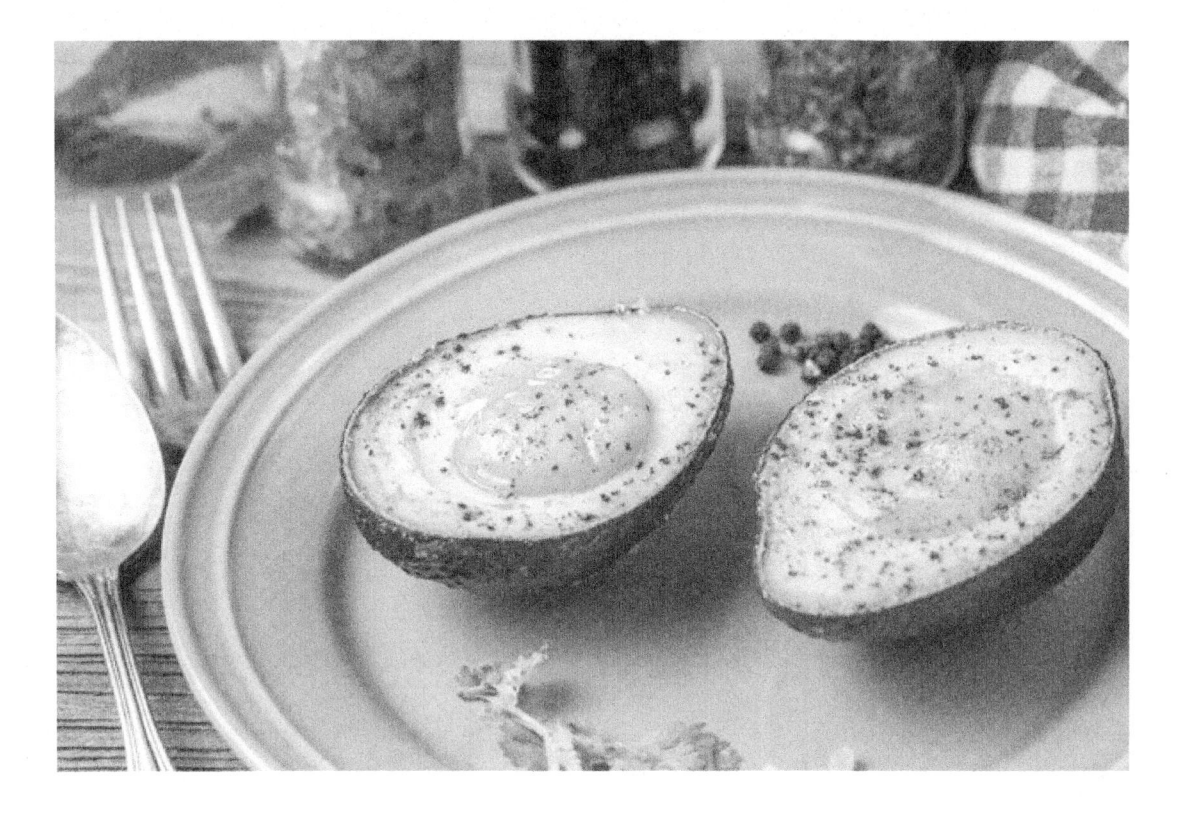

Again, I talked about stuffing vegetables with eggs to make a beautiful and healthy breakfast. Avocados are easy to work with; because once you remove the pit, you are automatically left with a nice big hole in the middle, ready to be filled with goodness. Then, you can create a scrambled egg mixture, or if you are ready to impress, you can also use fried sunny side up eggs to make it look extra beautiful.

Serving Size: 4

Cooking Time: 45 Minutes

Ingredients:

- 2 large avocados, pitted and cut in halves
- 4 large eggs
- Salt, pepper
- 4 slices cooked bacon
- Crumbled Feta cheese
- Lemon juice
- Unsalted butter

Instructions:

1) Get a pan ready, melt butter and cook 4 sunny side up eggs seasoned with salt and pepper.

2) Drizzle some lemon juice on the avocados so they do not become brownish.

3) Place one on each plate and once the egg is cooked, carefully place it in each avocado cavity. Complete with a slice of bacon, cut in half. And some feta cheese on top. Serve with a spoon.

Conclusion

This cookbook was about an amazingly simple ingredient: eggs. Eggs are a staple, as we established; you should always keep eggs in your refrigerator. Not only will you need to add eggs when you are baking, but you can also always default to an eggs-based meal any time of the day. Eggs do not necessarily mean breakfast, as we also established. They mean proteins, however, and no carbs, so excellent for many diets such as a keto diet.

Are you ready to learn more about eggs? Here it is.

It seems like eggs have been a forever versatile item. Apparently, chickens were brought to Europe over 500 BC. Then came eggs. Some other birds were also used for their eggs, such as quails, ostriches, ducks, and even pelicans! Back then, some of the eggs' shells were even crushed on plated to get rid of bad spirits.

France decided, in the seventeenth century, to introduce what seems the first attempt at scrambled eggs with some citrus juice, making it more like a lemon curd product. Then, from there, different uses of eggs began dried eggs, frozen eggs, eggs in a carton, and so on.

Now, if you are allergic or choose not to consume eggs, you can opt for somewhat satisfying alternatives. In baking, for example, substitute eggs by using tofu, cornstarch, or potato starch. You can go to a fruit way and add bananas and applesauce to give a moist texture. I also heard some people using chickpea puree; I personally never tried it.

If you are worried about your cholesterol levels mentioned before, using egg whites is a great idea. If you are picking up egg substitutes at the store or sign the egg whites after cracking eggs, you will get the benefit of the vitamins and minerals added. Fresh egg yolk is normally the one that contains all extra good stuff.

As always, if you have any health concerns, we beg you to consult a healthcare provider you trust.

We are concluding our cookbook about eggs here. We loved sharing, once again, our recipes, also our hearts and souls through them to you. It is our gift, and we hope you will always remember that eggs are an excellent source of proteins, and you can count on eggs to always provide you the taste and consistency you are looking for.

About the Author

Ivy's mission is to share her recipes with the world. Even though she is not a professional cook she has always had that flair toward cooking. Her hands create magic. She can make even the simplest recipe tastes superb. Everyone who has tried her food has astounding their compliments was what made her think about writing recipes.

She wanted everyone to have a taste of her creations aside from close family and friends. So, deciding to write recipes was her winning decision. She isn't interested in popularity, but how many people have her recipes reached and touched people. Each recipe in her cookbooks is special and has a special meaning in her life. This means that each recipe is created with attention and love. Every ingredient carefully picked, every combination tried and tested.

Her mission started on her birthday about 9 years ago, when her guests couldn't stop prizing the food on the table. The next thing she did was organizing an event where chefs from restaurants were tasting her recipes. This event gave her the courage to start spreading her recipes.

She has written many cookbooks and she is still working on more. There is no end in the art of cooking; all you need is inspiration, love, and dedication.

Author's Afterthoughts

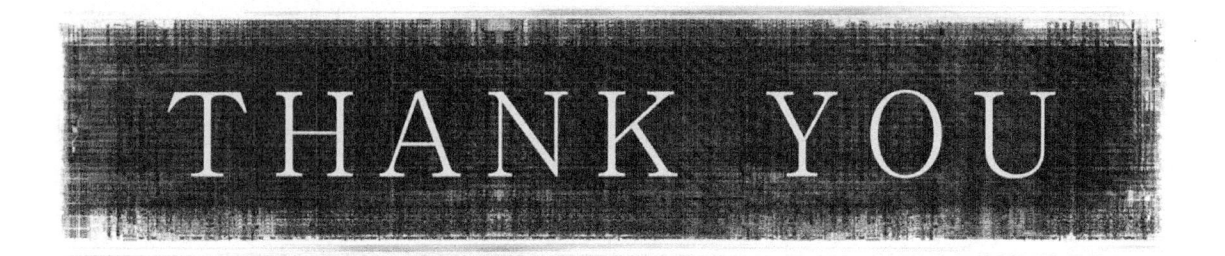

THANK YOU

I am thankful for downloading this book and taking the time to read it. I know that you have learned a lot and you had a great time reading it. Writing books is the best way to share the skills I have with your and the best tips too.

I know that there are many books and choosing my book is amazing. I am thankful that you stopped and took time to decide. You made a great decision and I am sure that you enjoyed it.

I will be even happier if you provide honest feedback about my book. Feedbacks helped by growing and they still do. They help me to choose better content and new ideas. So, maybe your feedback can trigger an idea for my next book.

Thank you again

Sincerely

Ivy Hope

Printed in Great Britain
by Amazon